YOUR KNOWLEDGE HAS VALUE

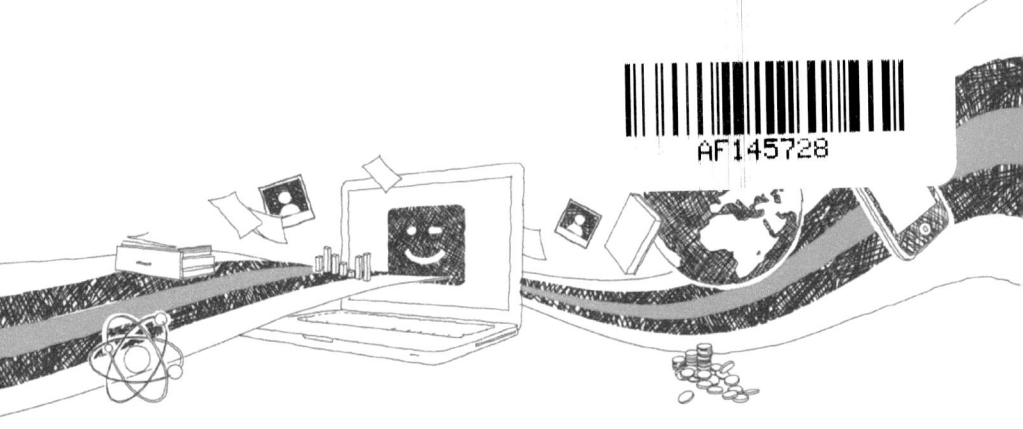

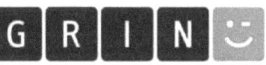

Bibliographic information published by the German National Library:

The German National Library lists this publication in the National Bibliography; detailed bibliographic data are available on the Internet at http://dnb.dnb.de .

Imprint:

Copyright © 2018 GRIN Verlag
Print and binding: Books on Demand GmbH, Norderstedt Germany
ISBN: 9783668797802

This book at GRIN:

https://www.grin.com/document/438250

Anthony Banyouko Ndah, Suinyuy Derrick Ngoran

Socio-Environmental Signatures of Cholera Epidemics in Douala - Cameroon

An assessment of community vulnerability and recommendations for effective response

GRIN Verlag

GRIN - Your knowledge has value

Since its foundation in 1998, GRIN has specialized in publishing academic texts by students, college teachers and other academics as e-book and printed book. The website www.grin.com is an ideal platform for presenting term papers, final papers, scientific essays, dissertations and specialist books.

Visit us on the internet:

http://www.grin.com/

http://www.facebook.com/grincom

http://www.twitter.com/grin_com

SOCIO-ENVIRONMENTAL SIGNATURES OF CHOLERA EPIDEMICS IN DOUALA - CAMEROON: AN ASSESSMENT OF COMMUNITY VULNERABILITY AND RECOMMENDATIONS FOR EFFECTIVE RESPONSE

(Second Edition)

ANTHONY BANYOUKO NDAH (M.Sc.), SUINYUY DERRICK NGORAN (M.Sc.)
Department of Geography and Development, and Environmental Studies
FASS, University Brunei Darussalam

SUMMARY

This study is an inquiry into the socio-epidemiological characteristics of sections of the Douala municipal metropolis in Cameroon in the face of recurrent and increasingly large cholera outbreaks in Cameroon. The purpose is to provide vital insights into the extent and nature of vulnerability of the populations to cholera outbreaks, as well as provide a leeway for the effective identification of maximum risk areas and vulnerable populations so as to tailor limited response resources efficiently and effectively. The study establishes the following:1). Contrary to the popular belief that in a cholera-endemic setting, the greatest burden is in the younger age groups (0-2 and 3-9), in the case of Douala, based on data of the last three epidemiological periods (2010, 2011 and 2012), the young adult / adult age groups (21-30 and 31–40 years) have been identified as the most vulnerable. 2). Concerning gender, males have been found to be far more vulnerable than females; 3). Social characteristics not commonly considered in public health strategies, including attitudes towards hygiene and sanitation, limited knowledge of diseases and cholera transmission mechanisms, as well as magico-religious beliefs on the origins of cholera, are possibly the dominant causes of high vulnerability to cholera and/or serve as major hindrances to effective mitigation; 4). Cholera risk factors such as slum settlements, lack of proper social amenities and services, for example, potable water, drainage, waste collection, hygiene and sanitation facilities, are generally spread throughout the Littoral Region and Douala in particular, though characterized by glaring unevenness constitute important risk facts but not direct causes of high vulnerability. Though there appears to be a direct relationship between the existence of risk factors and vulnerability, human attitudes and beliefs are the bridge linking these two concepts. Finally, an Integrated Cholera Management (ICM) framework has been proposed. This framework is intended to show the interconnected components of an ideal cholera management system in Cameroon.

1. INTRODUCTION

Cholera is a bacterial disease caused by *Vibrio cholerae*, which has been found to be native to coastal ecosystems. Vibrios, including *V. cholerae*, can be found in virtually any coastal water body, especially in the tropics and subtropics (Lipp et al. 2002). The virus is spread by fecal-oral transmission and causes a range of disease from asymptomatic or sub-clinical infection to severe dehydrating diarrhoea that can cause death within 6-12 hours, a limited period of time during which patients can lose more than 10% of their body weight in fluid losses, and adults can lose 20 litres or more (Weil 2012).

1.1. The state of global cholera epidemiology

The disease is believed to occur in epidemic proportions and become endemic in areas of the world where the 20th century innovations of clean water and latrine use are not yet realized such as in the poor parts of Southeast Asia especially in the Ganges Delta where 3-5 million cases are recorded each year (Weil 2012), as well as in Africa. Cholera is indeed a global health catastrophe, though the brunt of epidemic events and impacts are borne more by poor developing countries. Even in the poor countries, the disease affects different segments of population differentially, imposing a form of epidemiological segregation built along lines of poverty and social wellbeing. In Africa, a recent online article by Nossiter(2012)reported that a fierce cholera epidemic is spreading through the coastal slums of West Africa, killing hundreds and sickening many more in one of the worst regional outbreaks in years, made worse by an exceptionally heavy rainy season that flooded the sprawling shantytowns in Freetown and Conakry, the capitals of Sierra Leone and neighbouring Guinea. The same article goes further to point out that in both countries, about two-thirds of the population lack toilets, a potentially lethal threat in the rainy season because of the contamination of the water supply. In Asia, the case of Bangladesh in particular has received much media attention. Being reputed as the most densely populated country in the world, the capital city Dhaka is home to at least 15 million residents, most of who live in urban slums. Weil (2012) makes allusion to the fact that the great majority of cholera patients come from the urban slums, particularly Mirpur Slum and the major causes of cholera endemicity have been identified as: manipulation of water pipes through illegal piping which leads to sewage mixing with the water supply, failure by most people to boil or treat their water prior to usage, and the general belief that in Dhaka, diarrhea is a common and somewhat normalized fact of life. In yet another study by Sur et al. (2005), in Kolkata, the third largest city in India and one of the world's most densely populated cities, cholera remains a persistent scourge in the community of slum dwellers. The authors note that the study site, 0.7 square kilometres in size, was already in maps from 1856 as an impoverished residential area known as Narkeldanga, which encompasses what is known today as bustees, legally recognized and registered slums, characterized by narrow streets with little space between houses, intermittent piped municipal water supply shared by several households, one or two latrines and water taps, sewage collected in open gutters which overflow when it rains (Sur et al. 2005). An earlier study in cholera-endemic Bangladesh from 1966 to 1980 found out that cholera isage selective, most common between 5 and 9 years of age followed by children 1–5 years (Glass et al.1982); however, Sur et al. (2005) caution that despite this selectivity, no age groups is spared during a cholera outbreak, though the very young suffer most.The precise mechanisms and environmental interactions that give rise to increased numbers of *Vibrio cholerae* in an aquatic environment have yet to be fully understood, and this is coupled with the fact that it is not yet possible to construct mechanistic models for prediction of their presence and abundance with exquisite accuracy (Constantin de Magny et al. 2010). However, innovative studies in the field demonstrate how closely cholera is tied to environmental and hydrological factors and to weather patterns — all of which may lead to more frequent cholera outbreaks as the world warms (Lipp et al. 2002). As early as 1975, Kaneko et al. identified temperatures in the range of 25° to 30°C as well as favourable salinity levels of about 15‰ and the bloom of algae (copepods) to which have a positive effect on attachment of *V. cholera* as favourable

2

conditions for cholera emergence (Kaneko et al. 1975). Following in this direction, recent statistical models presented in a study by Louis et al (2003)provide a valuable understanding of the large-scale processes that dominate the ecology of *V.cholerae* by showing that seasonal pattern of occurrence of *V. cholera* was correlated with higher temperatures, indicating that there is a temperature threshold between 17 and 19°C, and the frequency of occurrence of *V. cholerae* is significantly greater at temperatures above 19°C and lower salinity levels between 2 and 14ppt, the optimal salinity being between 2 and 8 to 10ppt (Louis et al. 2003). Therefore, if *Vibrio cholera* is a free living occupant of aquatic environments, why then are some areas experiencing severe epidemic outbreaks year in year out, where as others record just a few cases from time to time? With this question in mind, while much research has focused on enhancing understanding of the environmental and ecological mechanisms which favour the thriving of the cholera-causing bacteria, social factors and attitudes in cholera endemic areas, which may contribute to high or low exposure of people to the deadly disease need equal consideration. Therefore, a sociological study of the attitudes and beliefs of people inhabiting an endemic zone can open a window into the vulnerability situation of the populations, as well as direct short term preventive measures which also save lives prior to the development of long term predictive and eradicative measures.

1.2. The State of Cholera epidemiology in Douala, Cameroon

Cholera in the Littoral Region of Cameroon, precisely in the city of Douala has become not just a public health crisis but a humanitarian disaster as well. Douala, the economic capital of Cameroon, located in the coastal plain of the Wouri Estuary on the Atlantic Ocean, also doubles as the capital of the Littoral Region is especially hard-hit. Infectious, emergent and re-emergent diseases have become important components in the medical vocabulary of the Littoral Region of Cameroon since recent times. Most of these diseases are related to water or the poor management of the water environment in Douala, and classified as very high degree of risk. Some of the most common include:food or waterborne diseases: bacterial and protozoan diarrhea, hepatitis A and E, and typhoid fever; vector-borne diseases: malaria and yellow fever; water contact disease: schistosomiasis; respiratory disease: meningococcal meningitis etc. The health situation in this area has therefore exceeded a normal public health challenge and can rightly be classified as a humanitarian crisis, given the frequent of yearly outbreaks. Of all the diseases listed on Table 1, Cholera and Malaria are the most dramatic and major causes of death, and therefore of greatest concern. But unlike malaria, a more silent health issue, which is known to be caused by the female anopheles mosquito, cholera is multi-causal, highly complex and characterize by spectacular outbreaks.

Table1. Summary of some major diseases in the Littoral Region (2010 – 2011)

No	Diseases	Number	
		Cases	**Deaths**
1	Cholera	**5669**	**9**
2	Malaria	11498	9
3	Meningitis	1	0
4	Yellow Fever	12	0
5	Measles	8	1
6	Acute Paralysis	2	0
7	Common Cold	476	0
8	Dracunculiasis	1	0
9	Gastrointestinal disorders	113	0
10	Trypanosomiasis	2	0
11	Hepatitis	17	0
12	Acute Diarrhoea	164	0

Note: the data was obtained from the Regional Delegation of Public Health, Douala in February 2011(Ndah,2011)

Cholera however stands out in the region which is endemic for the deadly bacterial infection since the arrival of the 7th pandemic of cholera in the Gulf of Guinea (Wouafo et al. 2007), with recorded epidemic outbreaks dating from 1971 through to present (Guévart et al. 2006; 2010). Outbreaks were observed to be occurring approximately after every two or three years during the dry season (Garrigue et al. 1986). Recent national trends point to a higher frequency of occurrence, with ever fluctuating mortality rates among the afflicted populations (Figure1).According to the Regional Delegation of Public Health, a total of 28 major epidemics have been recorded in Douala alone; the most deadly being those of 1971, 1983, 1991, 1996, 1998, 2004, 2005, 2010, 2011, with over a thousand cases each (Fouda 2012). A major outbreak was experienced in January 2004 and during which approximately 2924 cases and 46 deaths were reported in Cameroon from the 1st of January to the 9th of June 2004.In Douala, more than 500 cases of cholera were reported within seven weeks of the onset of the pandemic, leaving at least 13 people dead (Njoh 2010; Littoral Regional Delegation of Public Health, 2011). By the time the disease subsided, 6000 persons were reported infected and hundreds dead[1]. However, a lot of inconsistency remains in the data from different sources. During the short rainy season of March and April of the 2010 epidemiological year, cholera peaked with an average of 120 cases per week, followed by a number of peaks and troughs, and by September to mid-October the number of cases increased to more than 400 cases per week in Douala, according to the Littoral Regional Delegation of Public Health, in 2012.There was a sudden resurgence of the epidemic in Littoral region, particularly in Douala and the surrounding localities, with over 430 cases a week, in 2011 and by the 44th week of 2011, a cumulative 3,792 cases and 77 deaths were registered in Douala alone (International Federation of Red Cross and Red Crescent Societies 2012). Official figures however place the total number of cases in Douala at a staggering 5,463 reported cases between January and December 2011 with a case fatality rate of 1.92% (Littoral Regional Delegation of Public Health, 2012). By the 11th week of 2012, in the month of March, the Littoral Regional Delegation of Public Health officially reported 33 cases with a case fatality rate of 3.03%.The situation is presented in Figure 1 and Table 2 below. It is therefore clear that Cameroon in general and Douala in particular, like other regions of cholera endemicity, the disease does not disappear after an epidemic peak but returns in successive waves making it of great relevance the need to identify environmental or climate factors that may promote epidemics, thereby enhancing understanding of the dynamics of the disease.Thus, it becomes imperative to provide answers to the following questions: what causes periodic oscillations in cholera outbreaks, and why are some areas more prone to endemism? (Lipp et al., 2002). Some studies have attempted to establish the underlying causes of cholera endemicity in Douala. Guévart et al. (2006) have provided a comprehensive description of the environmental factors contributing to cholera endemicity in Douala. The natural location of Douala in the Cameroon estuary, an environment characterized by poor water circulation due to its low-lying nature, as well as high demographic and socio-economic pressures; the sandy clay soils which are poorly consolidated and facilitates the contamination of ground water; shallow dirty polluted foul-smelling groundwater; the presence of vast expanses of swamps, streams or drainage ditches, infested with Algae; high temperatures with low rainfall and drought during certain periods of the year, (Guévart et al., 2006) have cumulatively subjected Douala into a cholera endemic zone. Tatah et al. (2012), in a localized study in the Bepanda area, found out that 27.4% of the water samples were contaminated, with high isolation rates being obtained from streams (52.4%) and wells (29.8%). The number of isolates was significantly higher ($P < 0.05$) in the rainy season (35.5%), 23 (24%) O1 sero-group isolates were detected in streams and wells, whilst 64 (66.6%) were non-O1/non-O139, thus concluding that water sources, poor hygiene and sanitation were a major reservoir and cause of cholera endemicity in the area, as well as climatic influences (temperature and salinity).

---

[1]Posted online by Dickson Njoke on Monday, 20 September 2010. Available on:
http://newconceptsounds.com/2011/03/20/douala-ii-campaign-against-cholera/ accessed on 02/2011

4

Table 2. Total cases and deaths from cholera in the Littoral Region between 1996 and 2005

Year	Total Number of cases including imported cases/deaths	Reported Deaths	Case Fatality Rate (%)
1996	615	11	-
1997	1709	180	-
1998	4603	316	-
1999	326	35	-
2000	123	29	12.12
2001	259	7	2.7
2002	66	8	-
2003	207	36	-
2004	8005	137	-
2005	2847	110	3.86

Note: Cases notified to the World Health Organization (adapted from WHO 2004)

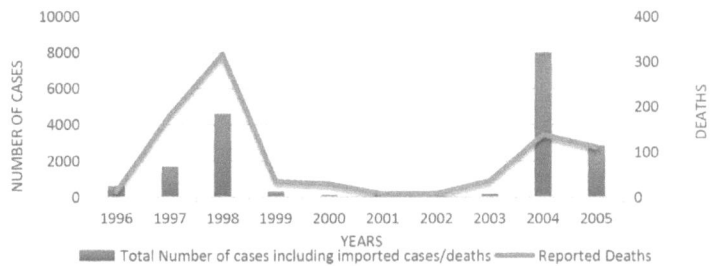

Figure 1: WHO-notified Cholera cases and deaths in Cameroon between 1996 and 2005

Similarly, a prospective study to investigate the extent of pollution and assess the scope of potential bacterial pathogens in the Douala lagoon has led to the finding that indiscriminate disposal of untreated wastes which are often heavily laden with sewage and the presence of potential bacterial agents such as *Bacteroidesfragilis, Pseudomonas aeruginosa, Aeromonashydrophila, Klebsiellapneumoniae* and *E. coli* in the Douala lagoon may pose a serious threat to the health and well being of users of the Lagoon (Tatah et al. 2008). This may constitute another potent cause of cholera epidemics in Douala. The important contribution of climatic variables such as temperature and associated changes in salinity, in the evolution and spread of cholera epidemics in Douala, have also been noted (Guévart et al., 2006; Tatah et al. 2012). The seasonality of cholera outbreaks also proves the point that climatic factors play a big role in the epidemicity and endemicity of the disease in Douala (Guévart et al. 2006). Characteristics specific to the city of Douala have also been identified as contributing to the frequent cholera outbreaks in the area. Most outbreaks begin in Bepanda, a slum built on a garbage dump in a swampy zone in the city of Douala; an over-crowded residential area which is the result of uncontrolled urbanization (Njoh 2010), with a population of about 11,000 people, who live without adequate access to clean water or basic sanitation facilities (Littoral Regional Delegation of Health 2011; Njoh 2010). Infrastructural lapses such as the absence of a good drainage or sewage disposal system in Douala, as well as the fact that the 8,000 wells in Douala (about 98% of all wells) are not protected and are located near latrines which definitely drain into them, have also been noted to constitute major risk factors, according to the head of mission of Medecins Sans Frontiers (MSF) in Cameroon, Max Antoine Grolleron (IRIN News, 2004)[2]. Shallow drains which pervade the entire city function as pathogen reservoirs and the use of water from these reservoirs for any

---

[2] www.irinnews.org/report.asp?reportID=39664 posted on 24 Feb 2004. Accessed on 02/2011

household activity are the most important risk factors that influence the spatial distribution of cholera in Douala (Guévart et al. 2006).

In previous studies, attempts to establish the causes of cholera epidemics in Douala have the general conclusion that coupled with its endemism in the area, economic poverty and poor living conditions, as well as the contamination of water systems with faecal matter and cholera-causing bacteriaare responsible for frequent outbreaks (Tatah et al. 2012; Peng et al. 2011; Fogwe & Ndifor 2010; Wouafo et al. 2007; Eneke-Takem et al. 2009). With this idea in mind, and with no solution to the poverty issue in the slum-infested city in the foreseeable future, public health authorities have resorted to the only reasonable course of action available to them based on the narrow techno-centric perspective common with medical practice – that is 'wait for the epidemic to strike and intervene with medication and awareness campaigns. In the management of the disease, a mirage of hope often clung upon by Cameroonian public health authorities as a measure of success in the fight against cholera is that the case fatality rate (CFR) of cholera, though still relatively high and constantly fluctuating, has been greatly reduced despite the skyrocketing number of cases in recent years (Figure 1). This has been attributed to the timely medical interventions during outbreaks, as well as free medical attention and treatment provided by health authorities. The primary treatment is rehydration, and in most patients oral rehydration is sufficient. In cases accompanied by severe vomiting, or dehydration that progresses to depressed consciousness, intravenous rehydration is required, while antibiotic treatment decreases the severity of disease and shortens the duration of symptoms (Weil 2012). This may however not last longer as the CFR risk increasing again with evidence of current resistance of the *Vibrio cholerae* to drugs.In a study by Garrigue et al. (1986) on the massive and systematic use of chemoprophylaxis which began in April 1983, it is revealed that during the 1984-1985 epidemic, 89.3% of the isolated strains were resistant to sulphamides, 87.5% to a sulfamethoxazole-trimethoprim combination and to the 0/129 disk, 55.3% to tetracycline, 91.1% to chloramphenicol, 73.2% to streptomycin and 94.6% to ampicillin. Unfortunately, these drugs have remained the major remedy used by medical authorities to combat outbreaks of cholera. Social issues stand prominent among the barriers to cholera prevention and control, leading to misinterpretations and misconceptions, especially during outbreaks in cholera-endemic regions. In the attempt to establish the underlying causes of high vulnerability of the populations of Douala to cholera, some studies have deviated from the focus on social infrastructural and environmental risk factors, and have cited social behavioural factors such as individual characteristics, societal norms and sources of health educational messages (Njoh 2010) as well as the reformation of urban tribes and persistence of traditional attitudes toward waste disposal and water use, which have not only led to high-risk behaviour but also created barriers to sanitation and hygiene (Wouafo et al. 2007). These however have unfortunately not been investigated intensively investigated and form the object of the present study. In this second edition, two major changes and updates have been made: firstly, the quality of maps and graphs have been improved. The maps have been re-made using GIS software METEOINFO. Secondly, a section on Integrated Cholera Management (ICM) has been added to the discussion.

2. MATERIALS AND METHODS
2.1. The Study area: The Douala sedimentary basin located in the Littoral Region of Cameroon, precisely in Wouri Division and has as major physical feature the Cameroon Estuary (Figure 2).

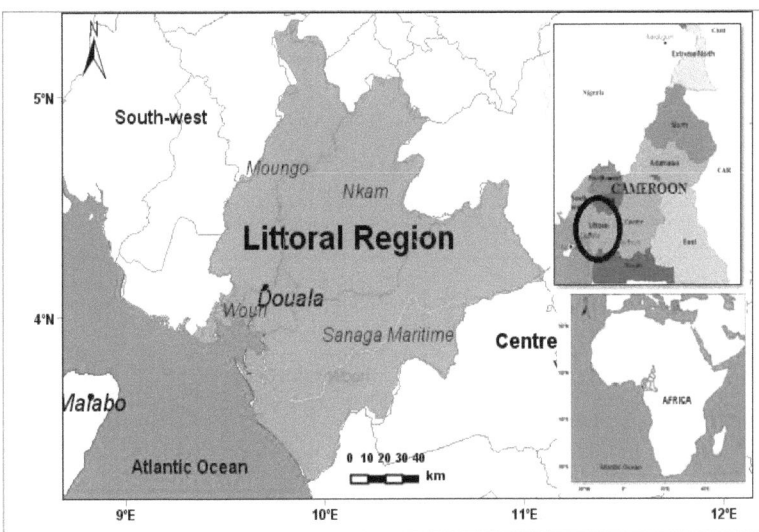

Figure 2. Map of the Littoral Region of Cameroon showing the Wouri Estuary

The map was produced with MeteoInfo 1.4.8. Shapefiles were derived from Statsilk, available at url: https://www.statsilk.com/maps/download-free-shapefile-maps#download-country-shapefile-maps

Geographically, Douala is located at latitude 4.1′ North and longitude 9.45′ East and covers a surface area of about 886 km² (Douala Urban Council 2011). This city of about 3.5 million inhabitants today, displays a nucleated settlement pattern (Nkem 2008), constituting the built-up area as well as the marine and coastal space is administered under the Wouri Division of the Littoral region of Cameroon. The Douala municipal area has grown on a typical marine and coastal space where the old barrier islands were colonised by the Bonanjo, Akwa, Deido, Bepanda Bassa, Bonamoussadi and the Bonaberi Districts, which today support high population densities (Asangwe 2006). Today, six sub-divisions make up Douala's administrative setup, each administered by a mayor, under the authority of a Divisional Officer, while a Governmental Delegate governs the metropolitan area under the Urban Council. Presently five of the six sub-divisions, which make up the Wouri Division are considered as strictly within the urban council and thus fall under the influence of the Government Delegate; areas whose jurisdiction is also claimed by the Divisional Officer (Douala Urban Council 2011), creating an avenue for conflicts of authority which strongly reflects in the poor management of the city. In addition to administrative lapses, the Douala area has the crucial problem of abundant aquatic terrain in the face of scarcity of land, which poses a serious challenge to coastal zone management, leading to environmental degradation as a result of the pursuit of urban spatial growth (Asangwe 2006).

Table 3. Subdivisions which makeup Douala in Wouri Division, Littoral Region of Cameroon and the major quarters

Sub Division	Major quarters
Douala 1	Bonanjo, Akwa
Douala 2	Youpwe, New Bell
Douala 3	Logbaba
Douala 4	Bonaberi, Bonasama
Douala 5	Bonamousadi, Makepe

The data presented in Table 3 was obtained from Douala Urban Council (Ndah, 2011)

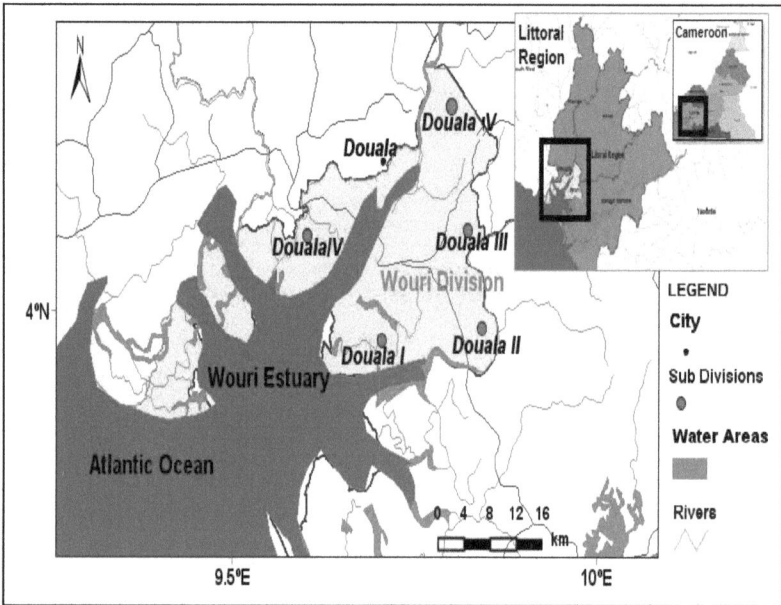

Figure 3. The location of Douala in Wouri Division and Administrative Subdivisions of mainland Douala (produced with MeteoInfo 1.4.8)
The map was produced with MeteoInfo 1.4.8. Shapefiles were derived from Statsilk, available at url: https://www.statsilk.com/maps/download-free-shapefile-maps#download-country-shapefile-maps

2.1.1. A brief historical perspective of the Study Area

In pre-colonial times, neighborhoods of the city of Douala,on the banks of the river Wouriwere ethnically based;Joss Plateau (today known as Bonanjo and located in Douala 1 subdivision), Akwa (currently located in Douala 5 subdivisions) and other villages were the basic parts of the city of Douala (MINUH 1983). At the end of the nineteenth century, the issue of coexistence between Europeans and Africans surfaced, and ledthe German colonial administration to impose its cruel urban policy based on racial segregation (Von Rhom Master Planfor the city of Douala) (MINUH 1983).This based on this plan:
- Joss plateau (now Bonanjo) was occupied by the German administration, the ideal position to control the port and dominate indigenous areas;
- Rapid acquisition of sufficient land to build a "tropical city healthy for Europeans";
- Creation of a safety zone of at least one kilometer wide which separates the colonial settlement from African quarters (Valley Bésséké);
- Programming new neighbourhoods for indigenous peoples led to the creation of a wide "free

8

zone" in the east of the city to accommodate the influx of migrants, people from other ethnic groups notably the Bamilekes, Ewondos, Yambassa, Banens, who moved in search of blue collar jobs (MINUH 1983). This area which included New-Bell (today located in Douala 2 subdivision), originally scheduled for resettlement of indigenous Dualas excluded from Joss plateau, later became the true focal point of the city with densities up to 400 inhabitants per km^2 since the 1950s (MINUH 1983). The city of Douala, as it is today, is divided into quarters, following along colonial lines, with Akwa and Bonanjo being the most important; Akwa being the center of Douala's nightlife and major commercial institutions, and Bonanjo its port and administration center (MINUH 2011). Bonanjo has remained a carefully planned area with gardens, squares and beautiful rows of trees, decorative street lighting and street furniture, though most structures are currently decaying due to inadequate care (MINUH 2011). Due to the overcrowding of New Bell, the initial settlement allocated to indigenous peoples by the German colonialists, new neighbourhoods grew and attached themselves to old one (MINUH 2011). This is the case of New Deido, Bépanda, Nylon or Nkolmintang (MINUH 2011). In recent years, the city has sprawled uncontrollably, extending beyond the traditional boundaries (Aeroport and Bassa Industrial Zones), with overflow to the North (Bépanda Quarter) and to the South-East (Madagascar Quarter) (MINUH 2011). However, these areas have continued to attract people from the rural communities because the promise of cheap and sometimes free land and affordable accommodation (mostly shacks) (MINUH 2011).The new quarters developing out of the old indigenous ones, today make up the subdivisions of Douala 2, 3 and 4, characterized by poor planning, broken roads, vast slum areas, chaotic constructions and commercially activities, very limited supply of water, sanitation and waste disposal facilities, and general low-lying, swampy and prone to seasonal floods (MINUH 2011).

Table 4. Population growth rate of Wouri Division and future projections

DIVISION	SUB DIVISION	POPULATION		GROWTH RATE	PROJECTION	
		1987	**1998**		**2005**	**2015**
	Douala 1	154.369	236.330	3.94	309.899	456.420
Wouri	Douala 2	152.304	246.800	4.49	335.543	520.385
	Douala 3	323.867	436.869	3.32	583.024	808.222
	Douala4	65.431	189.000	10.12	371.211	973.686
	Douala5	130.000	296.647	7.79	501.472	1.061.624
TOTAL		**825971**	**1432646**	**29.66**	**2101149**	**3900417**

According to the Littoral Department of Statistics and National Accounting, Wouri Division alone has a population density of 3830 inhabitants/km^2. Moreover, the population of Douala continues to grow at a rate of 3.4% higher than the national average of 2.9. This, however, varies a great deal between the different subdivisions which make up the Division (Table 4). This huge population has led to the "mushrooming" of industries, slums and squatter settlements which lack basic amenities such as clean water for drinking but have several shallow and polluted wells which are also closely located by pit latrines (Guevart et al. 2006; Peng et al. 2011).

3. DATA COLLECTION AND ANALYSIS

This stage of the study, which seeks to establish the sociological signatures of cholera as well as community vulnerability, investigates samples (households) from five of the six the sub-divisions which make up the Douala municipal area (Douala 1-5) (Table 5). Two main methods were utilized to collect data for this study namely questionnaires and interviews. Interviews were conducted with relevant officials at the Littoral Regional Delegation of Public Health, from where vital statistics on the total incidence of cholera in the region as well as data on the disparities in cholera vulnerability between age groups and gender, were obtained. Questionnaires, the major data collection tool for this study, were administered based on stratified random sampling techniques. The quarters and health districts constituted the major sample strata. A systematic sampling technique was utilized to derive the final sample population. The questionnaire which is of the structured open-ended type contains 10 questions, relating to the following broad sections:

  i. Family health status relating to cholera
  ii. Household water supply and treatment
  iii. Household refuse disposal habits
  iv. Susceptibility to floods
  v. Nature and quality of hygiene and sanitation facilities
  vi. Household knowledge on cholera contraction and spread
  vii. Household beliefs on the origin and spread of illnesses (cholera).

The sample of this study constitutes 1657 households drawn from five subdivisions (Douala 1 – 5).The average number of households per subdivision is 331 (approximately 20% of the households). The largest number of household samples was drawn from Douala 3 and 4, notably in the localities of Mabanda and Grand Hangar in the Bonaberi area (Table 5).

Table 5. Distribution of sampled households by Subdivision

SUB DIVISIONS	NUMBER OF HOUSEHOLDS	%
Douala 1	337	20.3
Douala 2	291	17.6
Douala 3	382	19.9
Douala 4	382	23.1
Douala 5	318	19.2
Total	1657	100.0

The results have been organized and presented in tables and graphs and simple percentages obtained using the popular spreadsheet application MS. Excel.

4. Results

4.1. General distribution of cholera cases in the Littoral Region by gender during 2010, 2011 and 2012 epidemiological years

Cholera in Douala, based on the analysis of the recent outbreaks of 2010, 2011 and 2012, has been observed to impact heavily on male than female members of the community. In 2010, out of a total of 392 cases registered, 218 were males while 174 were females. A similar but more dramatic scenario was experienced in 2011, whereby a total of 5653 cases were recorded, with males constituting 3321 case while females made up the rest, 2599. The data for 2012 epidemiological year though incomplete (January – May), shows a similar trend. Going by health districts, the number of male victims surpassed the female in all health districts except two health districts (Logbaba and Nylon), which had slightly higher numbers of female victims in 2010.

10

Table 6. Distribution of cholera cases by gender in the six Health Districts of Douala (data obtained form the Littoral Regional Delegation of Public Health in 2012)

HEALTH DISTRICTS	2010			2011			2012		
	Female	Male	Total	Female	Male	Total	Female	Male	TOTAL
BONASSAMA	22	46	68	301	401	702	0	20	20
CITE DES PALMIER	5	7	12	94	130	224	5	5	10
DEIDO	28	41	69	770	930	1,700	0	5	5
LOGBABA	28	16	44	88	162	250	0	0	0
NEW-BELL	53	77	130	473	624	1,097	1	10	11
NYLON	38	31	69	745	935	1,680	11	11	22
TOTAL	174	218	392	2,471	3182	5653	17	51	68
Percentage	44.39	55.61		43.71	56.29		25.00	75.00	

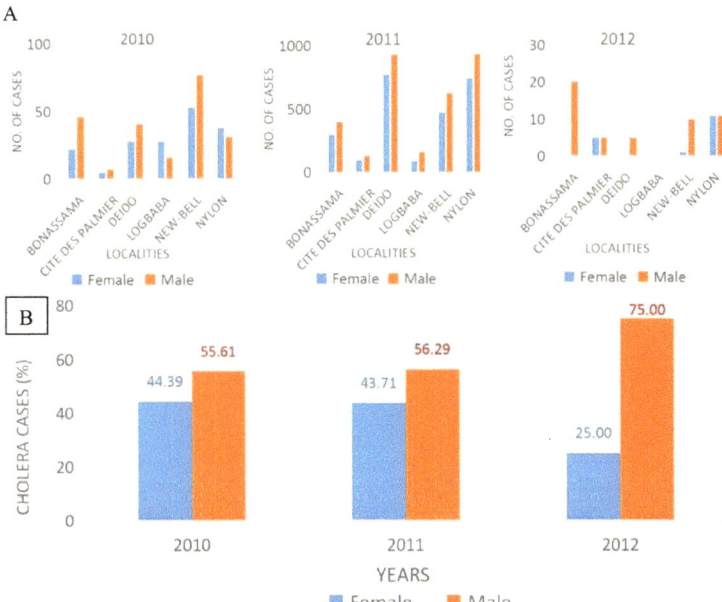

Figure 3. A. Number of cholera cases per health district and B. percentage distribution of cases by gender

The underlying reason for this gender disparity is currently not known and can only be speculated. However, based on field interviews and surveys, the most probable explanation for this variation may be that: though the population structure of Douala is slightly dominated by females, all economic activities are dominated by males especially in the informal sector (NIS 2005). This

11

sector employs the majority of young men who migrate from villages, mainly as street vendors and manual labourers. By moving from place to place, they become more exposed to cholera, especially coupled with the absence of public potable water facilities, forcing them to purchase water of doubtful sources and quality sold on the streets, or drink from exposed wells.

4.2. Distribution of Cholera cases in Littoral Region by Age-groups during the 2010, 2011 and 2012 Epidemiological Years

In the literature, Cholera has been said to be fairly age-selective, the brunt of its impacts falling heavily on the youthful age groups (0 - 10 years). However, as can be observed from the data presented here, obtained from the Littoral Regional Delegation of Public Health, the adult age groups, 20-30, 31–40 are the most vulnerable groups. Similarly, no reasons have been advanced for this disparity but the high mobility of these age groups compared to the others can be held accountable.

Table 7. Distribution of Cholera cases by age groups, 2010

Age groups	No. of cases	%	Cumulative %
>0 - 10	60	14.40	14.40
>10 - 20	61	14.60	28.90
>20 - 30	134	32.10	61.00
>30 - 40	76	18.20	79.20
>40 - 50	41	9.80	89.00
>50 - 60	25	6.00	95.00
>60 - 70	16	3.80	98.80
>70 - 80	5	1.20	100.00
Total	418	100.00	100.00

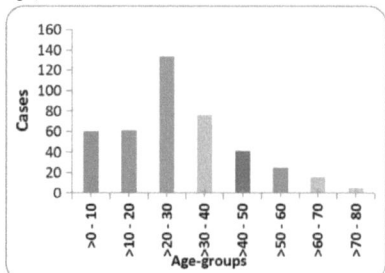

Figure 4. Cholera cases by age-groups - Year 2010

Table 8. Distribution of Cholera cases by age groups, 2011

Age groups	No.	%	Cumulative%
>0 - 10	708	12.10	12.10
>10 - 20	937	16.00	28.10
>20 - 30	1897	32.40	60.50
>30 - 40	1116	19.10	79.60
>40 - 50	596	10.20	89.70
>50 - 60	370	6.30	96.10
>60 - 70	137	2.30	98.40
>70 - 80	74	1.30	99.70
>80 - 90	18	0.30	100.0
>90	2	0.00	100.0
Total	5855	100.0	100.0

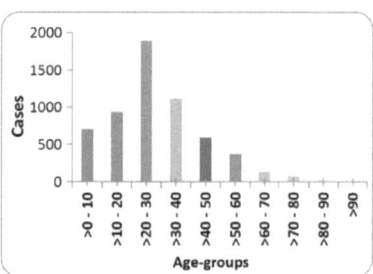

Figure 5. Cholera cases by age-groups –Year : 2011

Table 9. Distribution of cholera cases by age - 2012

Age groups	No.	%	Cumulative %
>0 - 10	1	3.10	3.10
>10 - 20	1	3.10	6.30
>20 - 30	7	21.90	28.10
>30 - 40	10	31.30	59.40
>40 - 50	5	15.60	75.00
>50 - 60	5	15.60	90.60
>60 - 70	2	6.30	96.90
>70 - 80	1	3.10	100.00
Total	32	100.0	100.00

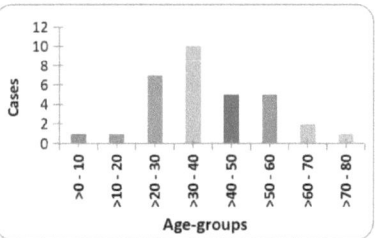

Figure 6. Cholera cases by age-groups–Year: 2012

In 2010, 2011 and 2012, the same age-group has been featuring prominently as the most cholera-susceptible group. The adult and young adult age groups are therefore most affected during recent cholera epidemics. Due to limited and the patchy nature of available data, an in-depth analysis of the incidence of cholera based on age

4.3. Sources and quality of water utilized for drinking and cooking and attitudes towards water treatment

Analysis of questionnaires reveals that 44% of all households utilize water from facilities of 'La Cameroonaise Des Eaux' (*CDE) for cooking and other domestic activities whereas 32.5% of the respondents use water from wells and 32% from springs (Table 10).

Table 10. Sources of water used for cooking and other domestic activities

SUBDIVISIONS	WELL		SPRING		*CDE		OTHERS	TOTAL	
	No.	%	No.	%	No.	%	No.	No.	%
Douala 1	43	12.8	1	0.3	232	69	60	349	100
Douala 2	69	23.8	1	0.3	202	70	18	319	100
Douala 3	123	37.6	18	5.5	97	30	89	362	100
Douala 4	291	76.4	1	0.3	59	16	30	351	100
Douala 5	9	2.9	5	1.6	130	42	164	308	100
TOTAL	535	32.5	26	1.6	720	44	361	1689	100

Table 11. DrinkingWater Sources in Douala

SUB DIVISIONS	WELLS		SPRINGS		CDE		OTHERS	TOTAL	
	No.	%	No.	%	No.	%	No.	No.	%
Douala 1	6	1.8	0	0	248	73.8	82	336	100
Douala 2	5	1.7	7	2.4	225	78.1	51	288	100
Douala 3	8	2.4	13	4	141	42.9	167	329	100
Douala 4	45	11.8	3	0.8	144	37.8	189	381	100
Douala 5	1	0.3	9	2.9	131	41.7	173	314	100
Total	65	3.9	32	1.9	889	53.9	661	1648	100

Note: *CDE (La Cameroonaise Des Eaux) is the main company supplying pipe borne (potable) water in Cameroon

Concerning drinking water, the households surveyed also stated a variety of sources from which they obtain water. The majority of households consumed pipe borne water supplied by CDE, the major water supply company, which is portable water (53.9%), followed by 3.9% from wells and 1.9% from springs. Other sources of water consumed include underground water and open water bodies, by a total of 661 households out of the total number surveyed. A clear disparity was observed between the surveyed subdivisions. In this case, in Douala 1 and 2 subdivisions, more than 70% of the households are served with pipe borne watersupplied by CDE, as opposed to 45% of the households of Douala 3, 4 and 5 (Table 11)

4.3.1. Household attitudes towards water treatment prior to consumption

In the case of water treatment, in general, only a few households treat their water prior to drinking, irrespective of the origin (35.4%), whereas as large as 64.6% of the respondents do not use any form of water treatment or purification before consumption. There was a significant difference between the subdivisions (0.016). In Douala 2 and 5, more than 70% of the households do not treat their water prior to consumption (Table 12).

Table 12. Attitudes towards water treatment prior to consumption

SUB DIVISIONS	YES	%	NO	%	Total	%
Douala 1	148	43.9	189	56.1	337	100
Douala 2	81	28.1	207	71.9	288	100
Douala 3	103	32	219	68	322	100
Douala 4	80	25.2	237	74.8	317	100
Douala 5	170	44.6	221	55.4	381	100
Total	582	35.4	94	64.6	1645	100

Note: Results presented in Table 12 are based on the question 'Do you treat your water prior to consumption?'

Results of this study therefore reveal thata large proportion of people in Douala consume water directly from shallow wells, springs and other exposed water sources, constituting a major risk factor. Water is particularly a problematic resource in Douala, in terms of its abundance and quality. Based on data obtained from the Littoral Regional Delegation of Habitat and Urban Planning (MINUH), the production and distribution of water is very limited and deficient, and the drinking water network which covers a little less than 40% of the city, remains to be developed and unevenly distributed. A reform of the water sector resulted in the privatization of the National Water Company of Cameroon (SNEC) and split into two companies namely: CAMWATER and La Camerounaise Des Eaux (CDE), responsible for marketing and distribution of water to end users. Despite this reform, the water supply network of the city remains old, inadequate and unsuitable, characterized by the regular interruptions in several neighbourhoods. Only 15% of households are subscribers to the official water network and most of them are from the wealthy classes, while 11% of households use a collective subscription. 1% of households are served with public taps. The vast majority of households (40%) are supplied by a tap water dealer or re-seller. Nearly 9% of households obtain their drinking water supplies from surface water sources (wells, springs, rainwater) (Ndah 2011).Based on the spatial analysis of the water network and the number of subscribers per sector distribution, large parts of the city are insufficiently covered by the drinking water network (MINUH 2011).

Consumption of water from wells and springs, especially if untreated, is very worrying.Previous studies in the area have shown that pollution evident from high concentrations of organic (up to 94.3 mg NO_3/l) fecal coliform and fecal streptococcus have been detected in the springs and bore wells (values of 2,311 and 1,500 cfu/100 ml, respectively); with pH ranging from 3.4–6.5, which is lower than the guidelines for drinking water (Eneke-Takem et al. 2009). The presence of bacterial agents like vibrio cholerea, sucrose fermenting and non sucrose fermenting organisms

14

have also been detected in well water utilized by the populations of Douala, posing great health threats in the study area (Peng et al. 2011);the most probable cause being the antagonistic location of wells by latrines, with a possible seepage of pollutants from the latrines into the wells as a result of the sedimentary nature of the Douala alluvial basin (Todd, 1980; Dumort, 1968 cited in Peng et al. 2011).

In addition, Douala generally suffers from flooding; due in part to the low-lying nature as well as its geographical locations on marshlands and/or near coastal areas and rivers; but flooding is also exacerbated by blocked waterways and drainage systems due to chaotic land development and constructions (Figure 2), and indiscriminate waste disposal. Flooding in Douala not only directly affect the physical life and property of the inhabitants of the area but also has enormous impact on water quality and the spread of cholera. This is because the flood waters wash the contents of the makeshift toilets and permanently putrefying mountains of garbage, into wells and homes, bringing along a wide variety of diseases, notably cholera. Former colonial areas (Douala 1, notably Bonanjo, formerly Jos Plateau, and Douala 5 – notably Akwa, Bonamousadi) are located on relatively higher ground and therefore suffers less intense flooding, coupled with better facilities such as road, storm drains and better planning

4.4. Beliefs and perceptions towards cholera epidemics
Though the inadequacy of potable water constitute important risk factor for cholera, beliefs and attitudes of the people towards the disease, personal hygiene and sanitation and environmental sanitation, and knowledge of the causes and spread of diseases, remain important determining factors for high or low vulnerability within all the sub divisions of Douala. In total, 75.3% of the households surveyed are of the opinion that there are no mystical reasons attached to the outbreak and spread of cholera epidemics, while a lesser but equally significant percentage of respondents attribute cholera epidemics to bad luck or witchcraft (24.7%). This latter category of people, in addition to being more vulnerable to cholera, also constitute an important risk factor to the entire municipality and even beyond because in such a cholera-endemic region and given the rapid rate of propagation of cholera, these people stand greater chance of contracting the disease and spreading it around. Going by subdivisions, Douala 2 and 4 had greater proportion of households which did not believe cholera had mystical origins (84.7%), as opposed to Douala 1 and 5, where a large percentage of respondents take an affirmative stance (40.5% and 41.2% respectively). Therefore, while there is a great need for education in all health districts, in order to initiate a change of mindset, this need is even greater in the latter subdivisions. Thus, with limited resources and man-power, available resources for the fight against cholera can be rationed, with Douala 1 and 5 receiving more hours of community health education and more community health workers than Douala 2, 3 and4.

Table 13. Household beliefs on the mystical origin of cholera

SUB DIVISIONS	YES		NO		TOTAL	
	No.	%	No.	%	No.	%
Douala 1	53	40.5	78	59.5	131	100
Douala 2	19	15.3	105	84.7	124	100
Douala 3	21	16.2	109	83.8	130	100
Douala 4	15	15.3	83	84.7	98	100
Douala 5	28	41.2	40	58.8	68	100
Total	136	24.7	415	75.3	551	100

Note: *Results presented in Table 13 are based on thebased on the question'Do you think the rampant cholera outbreaks in Douala might have mystical origins?'*

4.5. Level of community awareness of the mechanisms of diseases/cholera contraction

To the question of whether non-potable water and/or the poor management of the water environment was a major cause of morbidity in the Region, 96.7% of respondents thought that non-portable water and poor state of the water environment was the cause of numerous illnesses, whereas only 3.3% had the contrary view.

Table 14. Community awareness of the effects of the state of the water environment on diseases

SUB DIVISIONS	YES		NO		TOTAL	
	No.	%	No.	%	No.	%
Douala1	334	99.1	3	0.9	337	100
Douala 2	267	92.1	23	7.9	290	100
Douala3	305	94.4	18	5.6	323	100
Douala4	375	98.2	7	1.8	382	100
Douala5	313	99.1	3	0.9	316	100
Total	1594	96.7	54	3.3	1648	100

Note: Results presented in Table 14 are based on the question 'Do you think diseases could be caused by the poor state of the water environment?'

Data on the major diseases currently prevailing in Douala (Table 1) strongly attest to the fact that water is a critical resource in the city, not only because of its physical inadequacy but also notably because major diseases in Douala are related to water and the management of the aquatic environment (Ndah 2011). Therefore, as mentioned earlier, in a cholera endemic region, 3.3 % of the population spread across all the subdivisions, indulging in risky behaviour such as indiscriminate consumption of water may endanger an entire country.

Table 15. Community awareness of the contraction of cholera via drinking water sources

SUBDIVISION		YES		NO		TOTAL
	No.	%	No.	%	No.	%
Douala1	331	99.1	3	0.9	334	100
Douala 2	259	98.5	4	1.5	263	100
Douala3	213	81.6	48	18.4	261	100
Douala4	343	91.5	32	8.5	375	100
Douala5	305	97.8	7	2.2	312	100
Total	1451	93.9	94	6.1	1545	100

Note: Results presented in Table 15 are based on the question 'Do you think cholera could be caused by the consumption of non-portable water?

Similarly, when asked their opinion on how cholera in particular can be contracted, 93.9% of households mentioned unsafe water. However, in the specific case of cholera, the responses vary significantly between all the subdivisions. In Douala 3 and 4, an important proportion (18.4% and 8.5% respectively) of the households did not think cholera can be caused by the lack of potable water (Table 15).

Table 16. Households' knowledge of the spread of diseases via contaminated foodstuff and beverages

SUBDIVISIONS	YES		NO		TOTAL	
	No.	%	No.	%	No.	%
Douala 1	330	97.9	7	2.1	337	100
Douala 2	259	89.3	31	10.7	290	100
Douala 3	302	96.8	10	3.2	312	100
Douala 4	374	98.2	7	1.8	381	100
Douala 5	280	89.2	34	10.8	314	100
TOTAL	**1545**	**94.6**	**89**	**5.4**	**1634**	**100**

Note: Results presented in Table 16 are based on the question: Do you think diseases could be caused by the consumption of poorly conserved and unclean foods?

Table 17. Households' knowledge on the spread of cholera via contaminated foodstuff

SUBDIVISIONS	YES		NO		TOTAL	
	No.	%	No.	%	No.	%
Douala1	325	98.5	5	1.5	330	100
Douala 2	250	88.7	32	11.3	282	100
Douala3	232	89.2	28	10.8	260	100
Douala4	318	85.3	55	14.7	373	100
Douala5	252	97.7	6	2.3	258	100
TOTAL	**1377**	**91.6**	**126**	**8.4**	**1503**	**100**

Note: Results presented in Table 17 are based on the question: Do you think cholera could be caused by the consumption of poorly conserved/unclean foods?

Likewise, as expected, a large proportion of respondents (94.6%) think that unprotected, unwashed or contaminated foodstuff can cause diseases, whereas 5.4% believe the contrary (Table16). In the case of cholera, the majority of respondents are of the opinion that contaminated and unwashed foods could cause cholera (91.6%), as opposed to 8.4% who do not share the same opinion (Table 17). These later respondents constitute 126 people, out of the total sample population, which is a significant number in the prevailing condition of cholera endemicity.

4.6. Households' attitudes towards waste Disposal
Concerning waste disposal, 45% of households disposed of their waste in open pits around their homes. 44.6% of the households disposed their waste rightfully in HYSACAM[3] refuse dumps, while 6% and 3% respectively dispose of their wastes in open spaces and water bodies (swamps, marshlands, streams, etc) (Table 18). An important difference in attitudes of respondents towards waste disposal can be observed between the subdivisions. In Douala 1 for example, a larger proportion of households surveyed dispose of their waste in HYSACAM refuse disposal facilities (77%) whereas only 10.4 percent of households in Douala 4 dispose of their waste in or are served with HYSACAM facilities.

---

[3]*HYSACAM is the only company in charge of waste collection and management in Cameroon

Table 18. Modes of household waste disposal

SUB DIVISION	OPEN PITS		OPEN SPACES		*HYSACAM		WATER BODIES		ANY WHERE	TOTAL	
	No.	%	No.	%	No.	%	No.	%	No.	No.	%
Douala 1	30	20	0	0	114	77	0	0	3	147	100
Douala 2	19	24	1	0.7	56	70	0	0	5	81	100
Douala 3	51	51	9	9	34	34	2	2	8	104	100
Douala 4	125	74	22	13	18	10.6	1	0.6	4	170	100
Douala 5	35	44	1	1.2	36	45	0	0	4	76	100
TOTAL	260	45	33	6	258	44.6	3	0.5	24	578	100

Results of a statistical and demographic survey[4] carried out in Douala supports the data presented here, as it reveals that reveals that, at least 45 million kg of waste is produced every month in Douala, and each citizen produces on average 500 grams of organic liquid waste per day. The same survey mentions that garbage collection covers only 40%, meaning 750,000 tonnes of waste are collected per year, of the 2 million tonnes produced annually – not including industrial waste. Thus millions of tonnes have not been collected for years now, requiring that that efforts and capacities be doubled to meet the real needs of waste collection in the city of Douala. Therefore, in this area, a greater proportion of households (80.6%) dispose of their waste indiscriminately open pits (74%), open spaces (13%) and water bodies (0.6%) (Table18).

4.7. Nature and state of sanitary facilities/toilets

Results of the survey show that only 32.7% of toilets in all surveyed households are equipped with hygienic water evacuation systems. Analysis of household responses also points to the fact that, in general, 61.8% of toilets in households surveyed have an open evacuation systems that washes directly into the environment (61.8%).

Table 19. Availability of toilets with sanitary water evacuation systems

SUBDIVISIONS	YES		NO		Total	
	No.	%	No.	%	No.	%
Douala 1	191	54.7	158	45.3	349	100
Douala 2	89	27.9	230	72.1	319	100
Douala 3	98	27.1	264	72.9	362	100
Douala 4	60	17.1	291	82.9	351	100
Douala 5	114	37	194	63	308	100
TOTAL	552	32.7	1137	67.3	1689	100

[4] Accessed online at http://www.nl-aid.org/continent/sub-saharan-africa/cameroon-unauthorized-disposal-of-waste-to-blame-for-disease-outbreaks/ on 17/08/2012

Again, there is a difference in attitudes towards personal hygiene and nature of sanitation facilities between the subdivisions. Douala 3 and 4 has more toilets with open evacuation systems (80%); Douala 1, 2 and 5 have less than 55% collectively (Table 20). More than 70% of the toilets in Douala 2, 3 and 4 are without water flushing system, whereas, relatively more toilets in Douala 1 and 5 are equipped with sanitary water evacuation systems (Table 19). This is an especially worrying situation, giving the high water table in the area making it impossible to dig deep pit toilets, as well as the very close spatial proximity of dwellings, characteristic of slum area.

Table 20: Availability of toilets with an open evacuation system

SUB DIVISIONS	YES		NO		TOTAL	
	No.	%	No.	%	No.	%
Douala 1	160	46.1	187	53.9	347	100
Douala 2	120	38.7	190	61.3	310	100
Douala 3	291	81.1	68	18.9	359	100
Douala 4	297	84.6	54	15.4	351	100
Douala 5	164	53.9	140	46.1	304	100
TOTAL	1032	61.8	639	38.2	1671	100

The results of the questionnaires and field survey reveal that the state of sanitation facilities in the study area is deplorable. Large numbers of toilets notably in Douala 2, 3 and 4 characterized by vast expanses of slums, are known locally as 'toilettes sauvages' or 'makeshift toilets' with no running water system, and no system to empty or clean them, from which emanate a stench which permanently pollutes the local environment, and a harbour for flies and other insect-vectors of diseases. In some cases, based on field surveys, the toilets are constructed with zinc sheets or wood, usually above a water body or swamp, into which excrement is dumped directly, especially in Mabanda area in Bonasama health district (Douala 2) and Youpwe in New Bell health district (Douala 4). Sadly these same water bodies with such sanitary conditions are used for fishing and other domestic purposes.

5. CONCLUDING REMARKS

The results of this study have established that despite being an ailment generally contracted through the oral route, the mere in existence of potable water, limited sanitation and lack of conventional waste disposal facilities in Douala, though constitute important risk factors, are not in themselves sufficient justification for the high cholera-vulnerability observed in the region. This is because there exists cheap and simple methods of water treatment, food preservation and personal hygiene, which are just not practiced by numerous vulnerable populations for reasons which may be related to their level of health education, beliefs, ignorance. Thus, an understanding of the vulnerability status of the populations based on information of their knowledge of the causes and pathways of cholera contamination, local beliefs towards diseases, quality of life, attitudes towards personal hygiene and sanitation etc, will serve as an important step towards pinpointing the real causes of cholera vulnerability, and aid in the search for long term eradicative solutions. Thus, as appropriately stated by Shah: "with the environment changing, the disease on the move, and poverty still entrenched in many parts of the world, "cholera cannot be defeated by medicine alone," unless with "a new approach" (Shah 2011), and this includes a change in the perception of the disease. For 40 over years, the inability of Cameroonian public health authorities to provide long term eradicative solutions, coupled with the continuous reliance on short term ineffective and inefficient reactive measures in the face of such a major killer point to two main aspects:

1. The complexity of the *V. cholerae* brought about by its significant social, environmental and climatic associations have led to poor understanding of the disease, and in many ways, masked the underlying causes of the frequent cholera epidemics as well as reasons for its endemicity and vulnerability of the populations.

2. Ineffectiveness of the Public Health Management System in Cameroon and especially the limited consideration of social and behavioural factors which contribute to increasing community vulnerability to Cholera. Generally, cholera risk factors abound in the entire city of Douala, the Littoral Region, and in Cameroon in General. However, a glaring disparity in these risk factors can be observed within Douala, imposing an invisible but real boundary between high risk and low risk areas. The high risk areas which also correspond to high vulnerability areas, have recorded the highest number of cases during all outbreaks, and have been generally identified in Douala 2, 3 and 4 council areas, where as Douala 1 and 5 are relatively safer. The main reason for this difference in cholera risk include: better social amenities and improved hygiene and sanitation facilities, less susceptibility to serious flooding due to locational advantages, better planning and drainage facilities, and better waste disposal, collection and management facilities in Douala 1 and 5, following along colonial footpaths in these areas, as described previously. However, pockets of high vulnerability still exist within these relatively 'well served' and 'safer' subdivisions, due to the rapid increase in population and the development of slum conditions on the peripheries of clean and well planned quarters such as Bonanjo and Akwa in Douala 1 and 5 subdivisions. However, due to stricter and constant efforts by the municipality, the situation is somehow under control, thus preventing slum conditions from engulfing the whole area. The whole subdivisions of Douala 2, 3 and 4, characterized by physical signs of total abandonment and neglect on the part of city administration, has been almost completely transformed into vast expanses of slums.

Cholera being a highly infectious disease which can kill within an hour is different from other kinds of environmental disasters (physical or man-made) which tend to be more localized; a single case of Cholera in an area can result in city-wide or even nation-wide pandemic within days. Though the populations of Douala 1 and 5 are relatively less exposed to cholera risk factors, indicating at first glance that they are relatively less vulnerable to cholera than those of Douala 2, 3 and 4, cholera cannot be effectively brought under control along lines of high and low vulnerability in the same city. It is therefore highly deceptive to plan mitigation strategies for cholera epidemics on these bases. This is because it might result in a complete shift of resources to high vulnerability areas, thus overlooking the pockets of high vulnerability existing in relatively less vulnerable areas; as a common saying goes: 'a single case of cholera constitutes an epidemic'.

Thus, the initial idea to make an analysis of vulnerability based on different subdivisions the focus of this research has been dispelled. Instead, it seems more logical to attempt an understanding of specific factors that contribute to an increase in vulnerability within the whole area irrespective of internal disparities in risk factors. This can reduce the cost of fighting this humanitarian disaster by redirecting limited resources to directly tackle vulnerability factors, in this case, social and behavioural characteristics of the population. Therefore, understanding the sociological implication of cholera by analyzing the relationship between age/gender and cholera vulnerability; the attitudes and perceptions of people towards cholera, as well as their interactions with the environment, has led to the conclusion that though the physical conditions of Douala contribute immensely to the endemicity of cholera, frequent epidemics are accounted for by the poor treatment people inflict upon their environment and living spaces, especially through careless waste disposal, their unhygienic attitudes, deplorable sanitary facilities, poor knowledge of cholera transmission mechanisms, fetish and unorthodox beliefs about cholera, and a general feeling of nonchalance and ignorance on issues of health and healthy living. As mentioned earlier, the mere fact that people must consume water from wells for example, is a risk factor, but does not directly guarantee that they will contract cholera. Cholera epidemics generally breakout when they fail to apply cheap and affordable methods of water purification such as boiling and sieving, along with proper location and construction of their toilets in relation to homes and wells.

5.1. Governance Challenges in the face of recurrent cholera epidemics

This study has identified social and behavioural factors as major causes of high vulnerability, and recommends intensive and continuous city-wide education and awareness programs in order to initiate a change of mindset and attitudes of people living in high risk areas so as to reduce their vulnerability to Cholera. This should be followed by the use coercive measures to reinforce good attitudes in hygiene and sanitation through constant sanitary inspections in homes and neighbourhoods by health authorities and the punishment of defaulters through heavy fines; the 'carrot and stick approach'. It is strongly recommended that detailed environmental, climatic and micro-biological surveys be carried out in the study area, to establish the background environmental and climatic risk factors associated with cholera epidemics. With no intention to ignore the responsibility of the government and various decentralized entities, it is obvious that the Douala municipal government and the nation of Cameroon in general are not on the right track in setting the stage for the attainment of Millennium Development Goals (MDGs) as far as human health is concerned. The continuous use of antibiotics which the disease has been proven to become resistant to since the 1980s; the inability to provide basic social facilities such as public toilets and waste disposal/management infrastructure, inadequate provision of potable water, unplanned residential areas; the yearly reactive character of cholera-management efforts in a cholera endemic setting, clearly attest to the ineffectiveness of the national public health management system. Government failure can be accounted for by:

1. The complex nature of cholera due to its environmental, social and even cultural linkages, which requires concerted efforts by all stakeholders: governmental sectors, corporate, academics and all members of the community. This is simply not possible for now, due to the highly centralized political and administrative system existing in Cameroon. All management decisions (including health) must come from the central government based in the capital city, Yaounde, with little knowledge of the prevailing situation around the country, as well as limited interactions between different ministerial departments. The strong plea made here is therefore that despite the difficulties involved with changing such a system, political efforts should be made to decentralize the health sector so that regional health departments can make decisions and carry out actions irrespective of the dictates of ministerial bureaucrats in the capital city, far removed from the reality in the regions.

2. The management of health issues of the magnitude of cholera in Douala requires substantial financial resources. The funds available to the Douala municipality and the Regional Delegation of Public Health may not be sufficient, as claimed by public health authorities, but are sufficient to bring about a big improvement in the public health situation if put in effective use. That is, if diverted from the over-reliance on treatment and antibiotics and the creation of inefficient cholera management committees, to more effective preventive strategies through intensive outreach and education programs, in addition to the provision of basic sanitation facilities and policies to improve basic household hygiene through constant home inspections, proper urban planning and management. Therefore, due to limited resources, a sequential cholera management approach can be developed for the city of Douala, on vulnerability lines. Based on the effective identification of factors contributing to high vulnerability, vulnerable age groups, vulnerable gender, and vulnerable localities within all the subdivisions. Knowing where direct vulnerability lies, as well as the nature and causes of such vulnerability are important for the effective response to cholera hazards in the Douala area. Due to limited data, the analysis of the relationship between age/gender and cholera vulnerability is limited only to the most recent

outbreaks (2010, 2011 and 2012). A more detailed and continuous study is therefore recommended in this direction as well.

5.2. Opportunities for Integrated Cholera Management (ICM)

Based on the results of study by Ndah and Odihi (2018, under review), for the effective management and potential eradication of large cholera outbreaks in Cameroon, a four-stage conceptual framework was designed. In the first step, the underlying forcing mechanisms or driving factors of large cholera outbreaks are identified as natural global ocean-climatic phenomenon including El Nino Southern Oscillation (ENSO) and Pacific Decadal Oscillation (PDO). Therefore, by accurately predicting El Nino events and integrating such ENSO predictions, and associated changes in rainfall and temperature extremes into cholera management strategies, is the first step towards effective predictive response. Therefore, the national meteorological department must be fully and actively engaged in the ICM at this level.

Secondly, improved coastal water and watershed management via an integrated watershed approach to effective nutrients and sewage control could greatly reduce the risk of excessive nutrient enrichment and limit the likelihood for algal blooms and the rapid growth of V. *cholerae* in the aquatic environment. The key stakeholders here must include the municipal authority, municipal waste management services, manufacturing industries, farmers' unions, quarter-heads, law enforcement departments. Moreover, public education campaigns must be launched, to improve the awareness of roadside businesses, street vendors, households and in schools, towards waste disposal and domestic waste management.

Third, there is the urgent need to reduce the incidence of floods and flash floods through proper channelization of streams, widening of storm water drains, and proper urban management, could reduce the spread of V. *cholerae* and limit the contamination of wells and other sources of water used for drinking and washing. This is largely the responsibility of the municipal authority, who must work together with the hydro-meteorological services, survey and civil engineering departments, to ensure effective urban development.

Fourth, is the need to improve socio-environmental / living conditions especially in slums and other impoverished parts of the country via the provision of potable water, and hygiene / sanitation facilities such as public toilets to prevent open-air defaecation. Education and community awareness campaigns must also be given a high priority, in order to change the mentality of socio-cultural groups towards hygiene and sanitation. In this regard, the municipal and community authorities, and social services and school authorities must be actively involved in the integrated cholera management framework. Professional groups such as medical corps should be an important element of the system, but located at the base of framework, and mainly involved when rapid response is needed.

The integrated management framework should therefore be a research oriented management mechanism encompassing scientists, municipal authorities, policy makers and law-enforcement agencies. Fines and other forms of financial punishments must also be implemented, in order to ensure total compliance. This should constitute an important source of financing. However, the major source of financing must come directly from the municipal government through taxation of businesses and industries, in case of major cities with strong economies, and from the central government/resident contributions, in the case of smaller towns with weaker economies. These finances must be deposited directly into public bank accounts to avoid risks of embezzlement and mismanagement, while the money obtained from fines and other related charges must be reinvested into the integrated management framework.

22

Effective implementation of the ICM will facilitate the development of an early warning and response system for the fight against cholera; a system which will effectively reduce societal vulnerability, as well as improve response timing and action. This is however to be supported by a strong political will and adequate financial contributions for further research, the failure of which may stand as a major hindrance to the eradication of cholera epidemics in Douala in particular and Cameroon in general. International organizations such as WHO can intervene by imposing guidelines and deadlines on the national ministry of Public Health, geared towards reducing cholera epidemic outbreaks by a certain time frame.

REFERENCES

Asangwe, C.K. (2006). The Douala Coastal Lagoon Complex, Cameroon: Environmental Issues. Retrieved online at http://www.fig.net/pub/figpub/pub36/chapters/chapter_9.pdf accesses in 07/2010

Cameroon National Institute of Statistics (2005). National Population and Economic Census. Douala, Cameroon

Constantin de Magny, G., Long, W., Brown, C.W., Hood, R.R., Huq, A., Murtugudde, R., and Colwell, R.R. (2010). Predicting the Distribution of Vibrio spp. in the Chesapeake Bay: A Vibrio cholerae Case Study. EcoHealth, DOI: 10.1007/s10393-009-0273-6

Eneke-Takem, G., Chandrasekharam D., Ayonghe, S.N., Thambidurai, P. (2009). Pollution characteristics of alluvial groundwater from springs and bore wells in semi-urban informal settlements of Douala, Cameroon, Western Africa. Environ Earth Sci. DOI 10.1007/s12665-009-0342-8

Fogwe, Z.N. &Ndifor, F.C. (2010). Tropical City Milieux and Disease Infection: The Case of Douala, Cameroon J Hum Ecol, 30(2): 123-130

Fouda, B.A. (2012). Analyses situationnelle des determinants de santé en matiered'Eau, Hygiene, et Assainissement Douala in 2011 (Preliminary Report) Regional Delegation of Public Health, Littoral, Douala.

Garrigue, G.P, Ndayo, M., Sicard, J.M., Fonkoua, M.C., Lemao, G., Durand, J.P., Dodin A. (1986). Antibiotic resistance of strains of Vibrio choleraeeltor isolated in Douala (Cameroon). Bull Soc PatholExotFiliales. 79(3):305-12.

Guévart E, Noeske J, Gérémie SG, Fouda AB, Mouangue A, Manga B. (2010). Weather and cholera: epidemic in Douala, Cameroon in 2004. Med Trop (Mars), Aug; 70(4):407-8, French: PubMed PMID: 22368946.

Guévart E, Noeske J, Solle J, Essomba JM, Edjenguele M, Bita A, Mouangue A, Manga B. (2006). Factors contributing to endemic cholera in Douala, Cameroon [Article in French] Med Trop (Mars). 66(3):283-91.

International Federation of Red Cross and Red Crescent Societies (IFRC) Emergency appeal operation update Cameroon: Cholera Outbreak Emergency appeal n° MDRCM011 GLIDE n° EP-2011-000034-CMR Operation update n° 4 29 February, 2012. p. 757–770 Vol. 15, No. 4 0893-8512/02/

Lipp, E.K., Huq, A. and Colwell, R.R. (2002). Effects of Global Climate on Infectious Disease: the Cholera Model. Clinical Microbiology Reviews, Oct. 2002, p. 757–770 Vol. 15 No. 4 American Society for Microbiology. DOI: 10.1128/CMR.15.4.757–770.

Louis, V.R., Russek-Cohen, E. Choopun, N., Rivera, I.N.G., Gangle, B., Jiang, S.C., Rubin, A., Patz, J.A., Huq, A., and Colwell. R.R. (2003). Predictability of *Vibrio cholerae*in Chesapeake Bay. Applied And Environmental Microbiology, p.2773–2785 Vol.69, No. 5

MINUH (2011). Agenda 21 of the city of Douala: Ministere de l'Urbanisme et de l' Habitat: Government of Cameroon

MINUH (1983) Schema Directeur D'amenagementet de l'Urbanisme de Douala: RaportJustificatif et cartes. Projet Urbain FAC, Ministere de l'Urbanisme et de l' Habitat: Government of Cameroon

Ndah, A.B. (2011). Sustainable Development Challenges in Cameroon Estuarine complex and Opportunities for Integrated Management: Focus on the fisheries sector. Masters Thesis: Xiamen University, China

Ndah, A.B. & Odihi, J.O. (2018). The Epidemiological Cyclicity of Large Cholera Outbreaks in Cameroon and the Strong Signature of El Nino Southern Oscillation: Opportunities for Predictive /Eradicative Response. Journal of Population and Environment (Under review).

NIS [National Institute of Statistics] (2005) General population and economic census, Cameroon.
Njoh, M.E. (2010). The Cholera Epidemic and Barriers to Healthy Hygiene and Sanitation in Cameroon: A Protocol Study. Masters Thesis, Umea University: Sweden
Nkem, B.C. (2008). Evaluation of Stakeholder Involvement Towards a Comprehensive Reduction of Industrial Land Pollution around the Douala Metropolis, Cameroon, ENSPAC, Roskilde University
Nossiter, A. (2012). Cholera Epidemic Envelops Coastal Slums in West Africa Published in the NY Times on August 22. URL:http://www.nytimes.com/2012/08/23/world/africa/cholera-epidemic-envelops-coastal-slums-in-west-africa.html?_r=0 Accessed in Jan 2012
Peng, C., Wase, M.M., Mafany, NM., Epule, T.E. (2011). Well Water Quality and Public Health Implications: the Case of Four Neighbourhoods of the City of Douala Cameroon. Global Journal of Health Science Vol. 3, No. 2. doi:10.5539/gjhs.v3n2p75 url: www.ccsenet.org/gjhs
Shah, S. (2011). Climate's Strong Fingerprint in Global Cholera Outbreaks.Report of 17th Feb http://e360.yale.edu/feature/climat'sstrong_fingerprint__in_global_cholera_outbreaks/2371/
Sur, D., Deen, J.L., Manna, B., Niyogi, S.K., Deb, A.K., Kanungo, S., Sarkar, B.L., Kim, D.R., Danovaro-Holliday, M.C., Holliday, K., Gupta, V.K., Ali, M., von Seidlein, L., Clemens, J.D., Bhattacharya, S.K. (2005). The burden of cholera in the slums of Kolkata, India: data from a prospective, community based study. Arch Dis Child 2005; 90:1175–1181
Tatah, A.J.-F.K., Pulcherie, K.M.C., Mande, N.L. &Akum, N.H. (2012). Investigation of water sources as reservoirs of *Vibrio cholerae* in Bepanda, Douala and determination of physico-chemical factors maintaining its endemicity. Onderstepoort Journal of Veterinary Research 79(2), Art. #484, 1 page. http:// dx.doi.org/10.4102/ojvr. v79i2.484
Tatah, A.J-F.K., Oben, P.M., Mbivnjo, B.S., Ndip, L.M., Nkwelang, G., Ndip, R.N. (2008). Bacterial indicators of pollution of the Douala lagoon, Cameroon: Public health implications.African Health Sciences Vol 8 No 2, June; 8(2): 85-89
[WHO] WORLD Health Organization (2012) Cholera Country Profile: Cameroon, Global Task Force on Cholera Control; Last updated on 17 January2012

24

Wouafo, N., Noeske, J., Pouillot R., Ngandjio, A., Ejenguelé, G., Quilici, M-L. (2007). Environmental Determinants Associated with *v. Cholerae* in Douala, Cameroon; Centre Pasteur du Cameroon, CPC: Institut Pasteur; GTZ

Weil, A. (2012). Cholera in Bangaldesh MGH:Centre of Expertise in Global and Humaitarian Health, Sunday, March 25,.http://phsglobalhealth.blogspot.com/2012/03/cholera-in-bangaldesh-introduction-ana.html

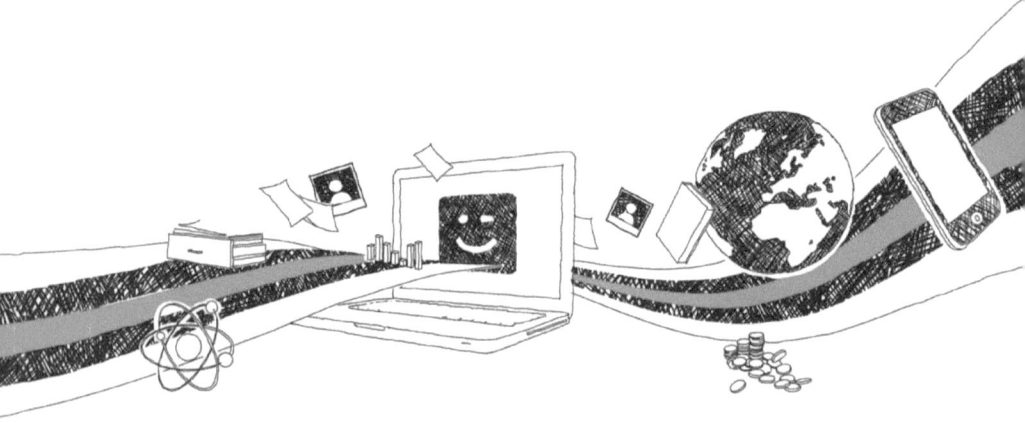
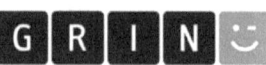